Use It, Nourish It, Keep It

(How to maintain your fitness and your health throughout Life)

By

Stanley W. Morey, Ph.D.

I Rose from the Ashes like a Phoenix

ACKNOWLEDGEMENT

I wish to thank my wife, Gery Morey for editing this manuscript. This book came to fruition thanks to her expertise. I also wish to thank my inspirations for this book Robby Robinson, a Masters Mr. Olympia winner, and Dr. Richard Baldwin a National caliber bodybuilding competitor, and Professor at Gulf Coast College who have maintained their fitness well into their 60's.

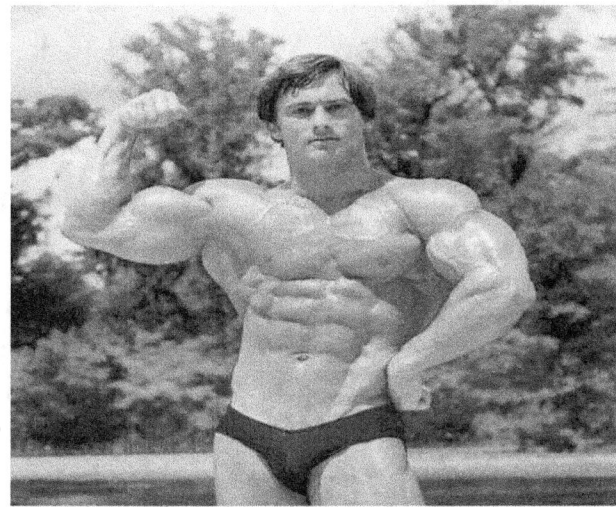

Dr. Baldwin in his 20's (top) and in the gym in his 60's (below)

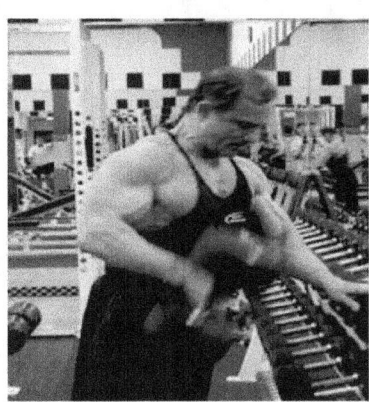

Prologue

In my early years I traveled the United States giving seminars to medical practitioners and athletes on nutrition and the digestive system, exercise and ergogenic aids. The two main goals of these seminars were to help athletes understand how these factors affect the body so they could develop an informed approach to improve their performance, and to educate them so they could avoid fraudulent claims when buying diet products, ergogenic aids, or nutritional supplements.

Recently I was diagnosed with multiple myeloma and decided to read over my extensive seminar notes to refresh my knowledge on health and fitness. That was when I realized that much of the information presented in my seminars would apply not only to athletes, but to anyone interested in maintaining their fitness throughout life. This epiphany was further enhanced when I thought of two friends - Robby Robinson (Masters Mr. Olympia) and Richard Baldwin (National Bodybuilding competitor). These two men competed as body builders in their earlier years and have maintained their bodies at that level well into their 60's. Of course not everyone wants to train to become a bodybuilder. But just like athletes in training, anyone can learn about diet and exercise to maintain any level of health and fitness they choose. So I decided to write this little book about how to retain fitness and practice a healthy lifestyle, no matter what the challenge.

I strongly believe you can maintain health and fitness throughout your life. The key is a clear understanding of how your body absorbs and uses nutrients, the role of proper exercise in keeping your body working well, and being an informed consumer when it comes to purchasing diet products and nutritional supplements.

Stanley W. Morey Ph.D.

INTRODUCTION

Have you ever wondered what to do in order to stay in excellent condition throughout life without living in the gym, running all day and reading about all the myriad diets available?

You do not aspire to be a bodybuilder with mounds of muscle that erupt with every move, nor a power lifter seeking to lift more and more weight, or a marathon runner, running from here to there. You just want to maintain an attractive, physically fit body throughout life – an aerobically fit, flexible, well balanced body that you fuel with sensible, healthy meals. You also want to avoid every new gimmick that purports to magically improve your health and fitness levels with little or no effort on your part. I hope to provide you with the information you need to make wise, informed decisions about your health and fitness. Let us explore the methods available to accomplish this goal and get you started on the road to a healthy, fit future.

1. CHAPTER ONE: PROGRESSIVE RESISTANCE EXERCISE

We will begin our journey by discussing different forms of exercise, their anaerobic/aerobic qualities and their ability to aid in maintaining your balance and flexibility throughout life. Because of my multiple myeloma, I developed nine spinal compression fractures, and have realized that even people without my diagnosis of cancer have problems with spinal compression, and need to avoid exercises that will initiate that problem. We will begin our tour by discussing Progressive Resistance Exercise or PRE.

Progressive Resistance Exercise or free weight training has been said to be superior to all other forms of training in producing results (Brooks, 1984; Berger, 1982). It can be subdivided into three types, isometric, isotonic, and isokinetic.

A. Isometric

In isometric exercise, the weight or resistance remains stationary. Increases in strength have been noted, but they are only limited to the specific joint angle being used. A dynamometer scale can be used to provide a readout of improvement or force applied. Isometric training is used by many strength athletes to overcome

"Sticking Points", which are the weakest point in a range of movement. Isometric training can be dangerous due to elevated systolic and diastolic blood pressure readings. People with high blood pressure should use caution when using this type of exercise.

B. **Isotonic**

In isotonic exercise, constant (free weights) are used. There is both a concentric factor (a shortening or positive movement of the muscle) and an eccentric factor (a lengthening or negative movement of the muscle). In this form of exercise there is variable resistance which means there is resistance over the entire range of movement. Using Nautilus equipment produces such resistance.

C. **Isokinetic**

In isokinetic exercise, accommodating resistance is used. In this form of exercise the rate of resistance and the speed of the movement are both controlled. Isokinetic exercise eliminates weak spots in the range of movement, uses expensive equipment, and does not provide room for incentive.

2. CHAPTER TWO: MUSCLE GROWTH

Increase in the size of a muscle fiber is termed **Hypertrophy**. It occurs primarily in the fast twitch fibers. The splitting of muscle fibers, termed **Hyperplasia,** is not thought to be the primary method of muscle growth. Below is a research study done in Sweden that seems to indicate that hyperplasia occurs, however, I find that this research, although interesting, does not substantiate hyperplasia.

Eur J Appl Physiol Occup Physiol. 1991;62(5):301-4.

Evidence of fiber hyperplasia in human skeletal muscles from healthy young men? A left-right comparison of the fiber number in whole anterior tibialis muscles.

Hypertrophy occurs due to the synthesis of cellular material, particularly the protein that constitutes the contractile elements. Myofibrils (muscle fibers) increase in size and number, with an increase of amino acid uptake. However, mitochondria (energy producing units in the cells that use oxygen) do not increase, therefore a large muscle is less aerobic (uses less oxygen, also called anaerobic).

PRE tends to selectively hypertrophy the fast twitch fibers, which are also more anaerobic. Since weight training is an anaerobic exercise, aerobic training must be added to your exercise routine.

In PRE or overload training:

Beginners should start with 10-12 repetitions of an exercise, while more advanced individuals should strive for 4-8 repetitions.

1. Muscles will only adapt to the load placed on them. Minimum weight gives minimum results.

2. Training can be more interesting resulting in maximum benefit.

3. Large muscle groups are trained before small ones.

4. Training is slow and deliberate.

5. Allows for adequate recovery time.

6. Research indicates that 60-80% loads are best.

We probably all have experienced some degree of muscle soreness when either coming off a lay-off, adding a new movement, or just starting our workout and exercise experience. It is probably one of the main reasons beginners quit training.

Muscle soreness is thought to be caused by connective tissue damage and muscle injury. Soreness is not something to be strived for in a workout. In order to relieve soreness, stretching, particularly static stretching, is best. You and your trainer should be aware of the benefits of stretching, and include them into your exercise experience.

Many people have asked if there is a difference in muscle Hypertrophy or force between a male and female. Actually, there is no difference between male and female muscles. Testosterone appears to be the primary difference which accounts for the greater hypertrophy in the male. I have been fortunate to help train world record holders, and national caliber female athletes, and have been able to test this theory of hormone differences between male/female competitors. I have noted that some women have naturally higher testosterone levels than some males.

Exercise causes a release of **Growth Hormone Releasing Substance,** which then causes the pituitary gland to release **Growth Hormone**. Growth hormone causes all cells to hypertrophy, which increases the metabolism of adipose/fat tissue, and conserves glycogen stores. Amino acid uptake remains elevated for 2-3 hours after training. Testosterone levels also increase and stay elevated for 2-3 hours following exercise.

However, what actually causes the work of hypertrophy, are hormone-like substances within the muscle called **Somatomedins.** They increase amino acid uptake and glucose uptake in skeletal muscle. Hypertrophied muscles exhibit large amounts of somatomedin.

Somatomedin is produced by the liver and various other cells, often in response to growth hormone release. Somatomedins are composed of 8 amino acid chains. They stimulate protein synthesis, RNA synthesis, amino acid uptake, and cartilage and muscle growth.

Strength is a factor that can be very difficult to define because leverage becomes an important issue. However, the standard definition of strength is the amount of force that a muscle can exert. The size of a muscle, or its cross section, is a major factor in strength. It has been found that the number of motor neurons involved, as well as the leverage, are prime factors in what we call strength. I have particularly noted this leverage advantage in superior dead lifters. All you have to do is study how these athletes are skeletally put together to see how they can be good dead lifters. They usually have long arms, short torsos, and very good grip strength.

3. CHAPTER THREE: WORKOUTS

We will now cover some of the most common methods employed in designing workouts.

A. Workout Schedules

1) Schedule a workout three times per week with a day rest in-between workouts. These are total body workouts and are usually scheduled either Mon, Wed, Fri or Tues, Thurs, Sat.

A weaknesses of this schedule is that it is hard to maintain focus and intensity for the duration of the workout. Overtraining, too little recovery time, and the fact that off-days do not provide caloric/metabolic levels are also possibilities. However, this is one of the most popular methods employed in fitness establishments.

2) Schedule your workouts six times per week with one day off. For example, Mon-Sat with Sun off.

This schedule incorporates a push-pull workout – (legs, chest, back); (shoulders, arms).
Three weaknesses in this schedule are overtraining, recovery time is less, and it is difficult to maintain intensity.

3) Schedule your workouts six times per week with one day off. (chest, back); (shoulders, arms); (legs). This provides a slight improvement.

4) Schedule your workouts over a period of four consecutive days- then take a day off. Repeat this pattern. For example:

M,T,W,Th,**Fri** Sat,Sun,M,T,**W,**Th,Fri,Sat,Sun
Bold days are off days. This provides a better workout result.

B. Modern Theory for Successful Workouts: Periodization and Recovery

    a) It has been noted by research that a muscle does not fully recover from a workout from 72-96 hours after intense exercise for max hypertrophy/strength.

    b) Workout should occur during daylight hours for maximum results. Research has indicated that sunlight (UV) light causes the body to produce testosterone.

    c) A protein meal should be eaten within 2-3 hours before an intense exercise session.

    d) Priority of muscle group intensity should be varied from primary to secondary treatment.

    e) Workouts should be varied for maximum interest, focus and intensity.

    f) Muscles should not be allowed to accommodate to exercise, which means you should vary workouts every 30 days.

    g) Maintain a high metabolic rate daily. Cross-train.

Periodization workouts have been developed by muscle physiologists studying strength/hypertrophy. You cannot train for both disciplines effectively, there appears to be a 20% drop in efficiency if attempted.

1. Load Cycle – Off-season (Mass)
   High number of sets
   Medium repetitions
   Moderate weight – based on an 80% single repetition.

2. Recovery Cycle – Active rest (transition Phase).
   Moderate number of sets
   High Repetitions – 8-10 repetitions
   Low Intensity – 60-70% of Maximum. (Heavy every 3 Weeks).

3. Peak or Competition Phase
   Moderate number of sets
   Medium number of repetitions
   High Intensity

4. Conditioning – Active rest
   Moderate number of sets
   High repetitions
   Low Intensity

Here is a schedule you can follow for a typical workout:

Chest (priority); Back (secondary)

Triceps (priority); Biceps (secondary)

Legs (priority)

Off

Off

Back (priority); Chest (secondary)

Shoulders (priority)

Biceps (priority); Triceps (secondary)

Legs (secondary)

3 days on, 2 days off cycle

12 weeks prior 5 days on, 1 day off

I have used this type of workout with many world-class athletes with great success. I have trained two world champion power lifters that were also world record holders, and a myriad of successful bodybuilders. I have also used this type of workout myself and found it to be enjoyable, particularly the change in workouts every 30 days.

4. CHAPTER 4: AEROBIC TRAINING

We have mentioned that PRE and/or weight training is not an aerobic exercise. Aerobic training should be included in your exercise regimen along with exercises that help or aid in balance and flexibility.

I will discuss my favorite aerobic, balance and flexibility exercises, which are Bicycling, Swimming, Tai Chi and Yoga.

A. Bicycling

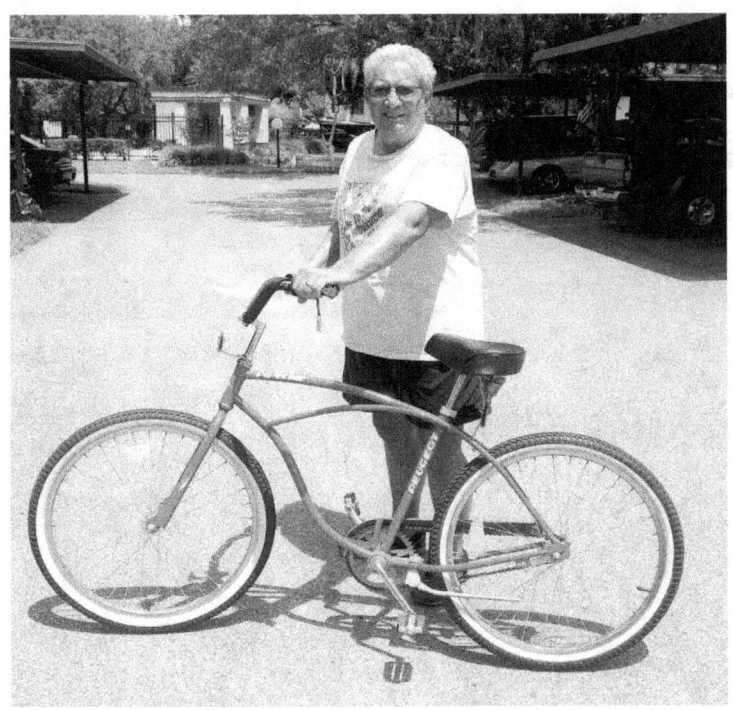

Author with Bicycle at 70 years young

I used bicycling as the aerobic part of my competitive bodybuilding training and have continued this exercise in my later years. I find bicycling to be enjoyable as it provides me with the ability to see my surroundings as I exercise. Besides being a very good aerobic exercise, it also helps to maintain balance.

Fortunately most areas have bicycle clubs that you can join which offer rides ranging from pleasurable to Century (100 mile rides). Even though the Century rides are exhausting they are an excellent aerobic exercise. Besides the bicycle clubs, there are many safe bicycling routes you can use as an individual i.e., Rails to Trails, which are converted railroad paths.

I still am able to ride my bicycle around my neighborhood for 1-2 miles, and this allows me to meet other people who also are riding their bicycles. Many retired athletes gravitate to bicycling to fuel their competitive spirits.

B. Swimming

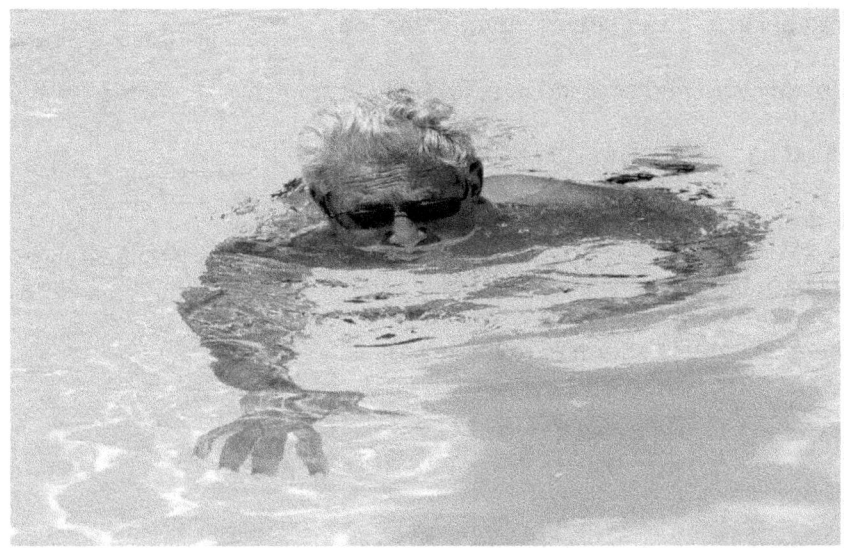

After my multiple myeloma diagnosis my inner ear was damaged which affected my balance. I found that swimming in the pool corrected my balance. I designed a program of swimming laps, and walking in the pool every day (living in sunny Florida allows me to do this). It is one of the most enjoyable aerobic exercises that I perform.

C. Tai Chi

Because of my impaired balance I was searching for some form of exercise that I could do. My wife had enrolled in a Tai Chi class, and told me how it helped her balance and joint flexability. She convinced me to try it, and was I surprised. It not only worked muscles I never knew I had, but my balance improved dramatically. Everyone should try this form of exercise, it is fun, and it works.

D. Yoga

If you are interested in improving your flexibility, this is the exercise for you. It is challenging at first, but you get more comfortable with the stretches as you progress. My wife does Yoga stretches at home and enjoys greater degrees of flexibility and well-being as a result. Yoga is becoming very popular, and is being offered in many spas, gyms, and Yoga clubs. Of course you should check with your doctor before beginning Yoga.

Because I have been unable to attend the local health club for fear of breaking bones, I have devised exercises to do at home such as pushups, chair dips, Hindu squats, pull-ups coupled with crunches, and leg raises. You can always find a way to exercise, and my book *"Quick and Easy Physical Fitness"* describes many of the exercises you can perform at home.

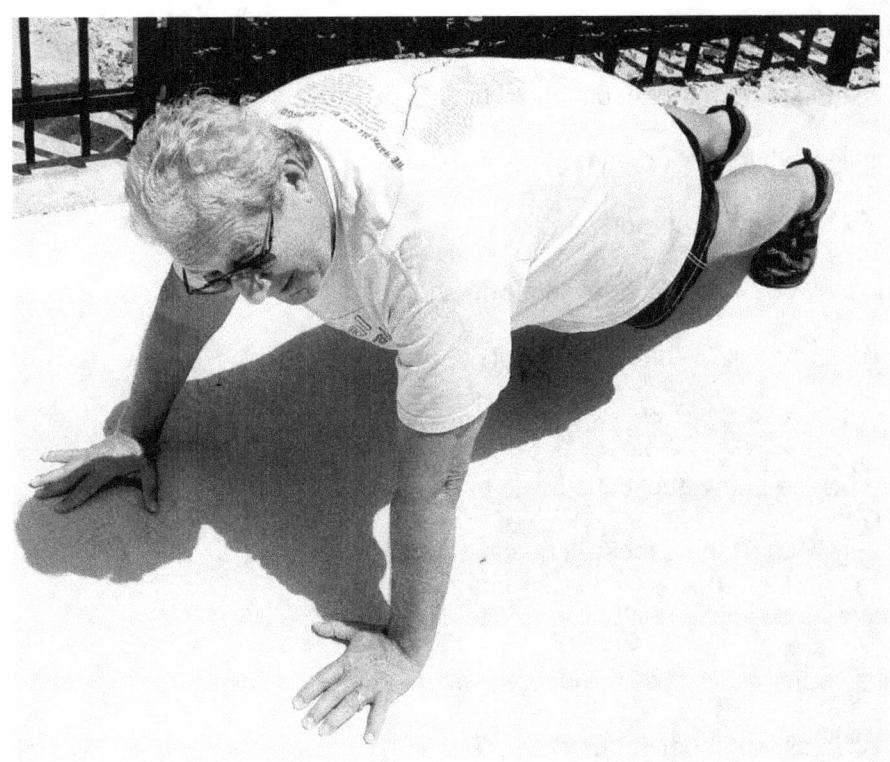

5. CHAPTER 5: DIET AND NUTRITION

Commented [SM1]:

A. Comparing Diets

We will now discuss an area that seems to bring a lot of controversy whenever it is brought up. Health and well-being are in the media both nationally and internationally. America, and the world, has become a health conscious society. A simple glance at almost any newspaper, magazine, or television amply underscores the increasing interest in health as an approach to daily living. Yet, with all of this attention from the media about health, nutrition and diet comes conflicting information and many of you are undoubtedly confused. What are carbohydrates, vitamins and minerals? What do they do? How do they fit in with the overall function of the bodies systems? What components of each make a health body?

These are just some of the many questions being asked by the lay person. Unfortunately, with all the exposure health and nutrition have received through best-selling diet books and television programs, there has been no attempt to explain the inter-relationship between health, nutrition, and proper diet. This section provides the individual with the background needed to understand how our food and drink directly effects every other aspect of body physiology and, by definition, the quality of life itself. My book, *"I Ate It, Now what?"* although at times technical should be a part of your library.

Yes! We are a health conscious society, but a very confused one. It is my goal to provide you with the knowledge to intelligently analyze information concerning your health, and to give you a framework of data to help you make good decisions toward a healthy and happy life.

This book will provide you with an intelligent and concise approach to health, diet and exercise. It will not offer you a miracle, or diet revolution but a sensible and practical approach to health.

It is with sincere hope that what is written on these pages will become a way of life, rather than a passing fancy. We will begin by comparing three of the most common diets, and discuss their positive attributes. The three most common diets are Low Carbohydrate (Atkins), Low Protein (Pritiken), and High Fiber Siegals). The table on the next page gives an overview of each of these diets.   Even though these diets are quite dissimilar, they all do work for weight loss. The problem is that diets usually cannot be maintained permanently, however, the Siegals Diet is one that I would recommend on an on-gong basis since fiber is always good for your digestive system. I have advocated the use of fiber in my Book, *"Nutrifitness"*.In order to continue our discussion on nutrition and diet, we must discuss what type of diet we should eat according to our digestive enzymes and systems. In our modern world, most people would class us as omnivores that can basically eat anything. They would be wrong. Let us examine our heritage.

COMPARISON OF THREE DIETS

PREMISE		
Low Carbohydrate	Low Protein	High Fiber
Obesity is caused by the ingestion of excess carbohydrate (over 60mg) or to a carbohydrate intolerance	Animal Protein is consumed in too great a quantity, is deleterious and contains too much saturated fat.	Lack of fiber is a deficiency that leads to obesity, constipation, and other ailments. In addition, mounting evidence associates low-fiber diets with heart disease, Colon and rectal cancer
GOOD POINTS		
Atkins	Pritiken	Siegals
Provides the dieter with a "satiated" or "full" feeling and is effective in short –term weight loss. The diet is simple to follow since the American diet is basically a meat diet	This diet eliminates meat, reduces fat consumption, and contains adequate fiber. Weight loss is good and energy levels remain high.	Diet is well-balanced, produces a "full" effect and eliminates the common digestive ailments prevalent in America. Weight loss is permanent and the diet is simple. Bowel movements will become regular, thus removing the large amounts of fats, calories, and toxic waste prior to absorption.

B. Diets and Our Heritage

In order to discuss our nutrition, we must decide what we are as to food habits (diet). The basic groups are: Herbivores that eat grains, Omnivores that eat everything, Carnivores that eat meat, and Insectivores (fruitivores) that each fruits, vegetables, insects, and eggs. In current society, we are considered omnivores, since man eats a wide variety of food. In actuality, our closest evolutionary relatives are the primates which are fruitivores. A careful study of our digestive system with its associated enzymes indicates that we are also suited to a fruitivorous diet. The digestive system is covered in my book, "*I Ate It Now What?*". We are one of the few animals that cannot complete the conversion to vitamin C because we lack L. Gulonolactone Oxidase (GULO) which is the last step for the synthesis of vitamin C. Fortunately, our ancestors lived surrounded by fruits and vegetables containing vitamin C, this constant source of vitamin C allowed them to avoid being an evolutionary dead end.

C. What is Food?

With that in mind, we will investigate what we call food. What is food? Food is any substance taken into the body to yield energy, build tissue, and regulate body processes. My books, *"I Ate It, Now What?"* And *"Nutrifitness"* describe food in much detail. Any amount of food, beyond what the body requires for these functions, is stored as reserve energy or fat. You are probably familiar with many different kinds of food just from your own diet. All foods consist of various combinations of the following basic nutrients: water (H_2O), proteins, carbohydrates, fats (lipids), vitamins, and minerals. We will examine each of these basic nutrients to discover what they are and how the function in our bodies.

Water: The human body needs water to function properly. Two-thirds of what we consume is water, 40-60% of our body is water, and 65-75% of our muscle is composed of water. A human can survive up to 30 days without carbohydrates, protein, or fat, but will die within 6 days without water. Water serves as: a transport system, a medium for chemical reactions, a heat stabilizer, and a lubricant for joints. The more muscle an individual has, the more stored water is found. The more fat your body contains, the less

water it contains. Prior to initiating exercise (within 2 hours), 13-

17oz. of fluid should be ingested. The following liquids should be

avoided because they have a diuretic effect: coffee, tea, cola,

alcohol.

Protein: Protein is composed of carbon, hydrogen, oxygen,

nitrogen, and usually sulfur, and makes up about 3/4ths of the dry

body weight. It is found in the cells of all animals and plants, and

is used primarily for repair and replacement. Protein is involved in:

structural components, enzymes, hormones, transport of oxygen

(hemoglobin), muscular contraction, genes and hereditary factors,

and antibodies. Proteins are constructed or made up of units

called amino acids with the following structure:

$$R-\underset{\underset{NH_2}{|}}{\overset{\overset{H}{|}}{C}}-C\underset{OH}{\overset{O}{\diagup}}$$

Amino Acid

C = Carbon O = Oxygen H = Hydrogen N = Nitrogen R = Variable Unit

25

Amino Acids are derived from protein breakdown in the digestive tract, and the continuing metabolism of the cells. The major role of amino acids is to serve as a precursor for the production of structural proteins. Non-essential amino acids are those that can be synthesized or made by the body, while essential amino acids are those that cannot be synthesized. There are 10 essential amino acids. In the course of evolution, the animal organism lost the ability to synthesize the carbon chain of certain amino acids. These must therefore be provided in the diet.

The essential amino acids are: **M**ethionine, **A**rginine, **T**ryptophan, **T**hreonine, **H**istidine, **I**soleucine, **L**eucine, **L**ysine, **V**aline, and **P**henylalanine. One easy way to learn the essential amino acids is by the mnemonic device I learned in a Biochemistry class:

Matt Hill VP

Complete proteins contain all the essential amino acids, and are primarily derived from animal sources. These sources include milk, fish, meat, poultry and eggs. Incomplete proteins are usually vegetable in origin, they do not contain all the essential amino acids, and include vegetables, nuts, grains, and fruit.

In response to an amino acid deficiency in the diet, the tissues do not make proteins lacking in that particular amino acid, but simply make less protein. However, the essential amino acids are not more important than the non-essential ones. In fact, the non-essential amino acids may play greater roles in metabolism. A good example is the amino acid glutamic acid which has many metabolic roles. It is quickly diminished during exercise and should be supplemented.

The liver plays a major role in protein metabolism. It is here that amino acids are converted for use in building proteins. The **transaminase** enzymes play a major role in this process. During increased protein synthesis, the transaminase levels increase measured in your blood levels as **(SGOT).** Transmethylation, occurring in the liver, is the transferal of methyl groups (CH_3). These groups are quite important in fat metabolism. Methionine is an example of an amino acid important in the process of transmethylation. The reaction that takes place is unique, and its actual method is unknown. The enzyme involved in carrying out this reaction is called the "Magic enzyme". Dietary methionine

supplies most of the methyl groups in mammals. Vitamin B₆ is
also important in amino acid conversions in the liver.

There are two major states of nitrogen balance in the body.
Positive nitrogen balance where the intake of protein is greater
than its breakdown through degradation, and negative nitrogen
balance where the intake of protein is less than the output.

There are several steps in the digestion of proteins:

 1) Protein is broken down into smaller diffusible units which may
be absorbed from the intestine.

 2) The stomach has an acid ph of 2-3, and it is in this environment
that proteins are broken down in polypeptides (smaller units).

 3) Peptide bonds are what link amino acids to form proteins. It is
these bonds that are broken when proteins break down to form
amino acids.

Peptide Bond
A molecule of water is removed from two
glycine amino acids to form a peptide bond.

4) Two enzymes present in the small intestine - pancreatic enzymes and mucosal enzymes - break down polypeptides and ultimately free amino acids. Milk protein and egg white protein can be absorbed directly, and can cause sensitization or an allergic reaction.

5) Time of absorption (lab) is15min-50min In order for absorption to occur, B_6 and Mn^{++} must be present. Liquid amino acids are absorbed much quicker than tablets or powders, 85-100% in 5 minutes.

6) Amino acid tablets demonstrate poor absorption. In 5 minutes less than 10% is absorbed, and less than 25% is ever absorbed. There is no storage form for excess protein intake. The excess protein is either excreted, converted to fat or glycogen, or used for energy. Muscles cells are constantly synthesizing new protein, the process is rapid and uses the free amino acid pool. An average 70 kg man synthesizes and degrades 400 grams of protein per day. The normal diet provides 160 grams of amino acids/day, and there are about 30 grams of free amino acids present in body fluids.

Below is listed daily protein requirements. The numbers are accurate to within +/- 10%.

1) The average person needs 0.36g/lb. therefore a 200 lb. individual would require 72 g of protein/day.

2) An active/endurance individual needs 0.63g/lb, so a 200 lb. individual would require 126g of protein/day.

3) A bodybuilder needs 0.9g/lb. Therefore a 200 lb. bodybuilder would require 180g/day.

The average American consumes 2-3 times the required amount of protein. Too much protein is deleterious because it is not an efficient energy source, and can impair kidney function and cause nephritis, dehydration, loss of appetite and diarrhea. In the lab, 1 gram of protein provides 4 calories. In actuality it only provides 70-75% of that due to what is termed **Specific Dynamic Action (SDA)**. This is the reason a high protein diet works so well in losing weight.

Protein in food and supplements is rated using the following methods:

Protein Efficiency Ratio (PER)
Casein (standard)   1.0
Soy isolate   2.5
Milk-Egg   2.5
Collagen   Less than 1.0
Egg   3.7
Whey   4.3

Completeness/Biologic Value (BV)
Whey   104%
Eggs   100%
Fish/poultry   70%
Meat   69%
Milk   60%
Rice   56%
Potato   34%

The branched chain or free form amino acids have no known role in mammalian metabolism, and they are part of the essential amino acids. The branched chain amino acids (Leucine, Isoleucine, and Valine) are involved in methylation and fat metabolism. However, if already taken in the diet, why should they be supplemented? However, these products are on every store shelf that sells vitamins. Protein should comprise approximately 15-20% of the mammalian diet.

Carbohydrates: We finally get to a passion of mine. The human body is a **Carbohydrate Machine.** Its fuel is carbohydrates. Carbohydrates are composed of carbon, hydrogen, and oxygen, and they are stored as **glycogen** in the body. There are 275g of carbs stored in muscle tissue, 100-120g in the liver, 15-20g in the blood, and 375-475g stored in other tissues. Carbohydrates provide 4 calories/gram, with an SDA of only 6%. Two forms of carbohydrates are **monosaccharide's,** which are simple sugars such as those found in fruits, and **oligosacharrides** which are double sugars. Three oligosacharrides are: 1) Sucrose – approximately 25% of your total ingested carbohydrate.

 2) Lactose – milk sugar – Blacks, African-Americans about 85% and a large percentage of whites cannot utilize lactose due to the enzyme lactase being absent. Can cause varying amount of allergic reaction and gastric distress. 3) Maltose – negligible in the diet. Beer is a good source of maltose. A third type of carbohydrate are the **polysaccharides** which are composed of many sugar units such as starches, cellulose, and glycogen. Carbohydrates should comprise at least 50% of a person's intake, however, we take in less than 30% in today's diet. Unfortunately,

Americans consume 80% of their carbohydrate intake as refined sugars. The world consumption of sugar in the 1600's was about 129 lb. /yr. Today the average person consumes greater than 100lb of sugar/yr. Carbohydrates are protein sparing, a primer for fat metabolism, and fuel for the central nervous system. 60-70% of the diet should consist of carbohydrates. Low carbohydrate diets utilize protein for energy, and *fat is conserved*. The Tarahumara Indians of South America eat a diet that consists primarily of complex carbohydrates. They are capable of extraordinary physical workloads such as 150-200 mile non-stop runs.

Fats and Lipids: Fats and lipids, are a highly misunderstood area of nutrition and diet. They are composed of carbon, hydrogen, and oxygen. These are linked together by fatty acids and contain large amounts of hydrogen. They are a source of potential energy, they serve as protection, and they are a source of insulation. In a normal adult male body, about 110,000 kcal are stored as fat energy, 1500 kcal are stored in muscle tissue, and 400kcal are stored in the liver.

There are three categories of fats – simple fats, saturated fats, and unsaturated fats.

Simple Fats are also called Triglycerides. About 99% of the stored fats in the body are triglycerides.

Saturated Fats are hydrogenated (the chemical bonds are saturated with hydrogen) and are extremely hard to breakdown. Animal sources such as meat and chicken are high in saturated fats, and they are solid at room temperature (margarine) The most abundant saturated fat in commercial use is palmitic or palm oil.

Unsaturated Fats have a lower melting point than other fats. They break down easily and liquefy at room temperature. They contain essential fatty acids which are:

   a) linoleic – contains two double bonds

   b) linolenic–contains 3 double bonds

   c) arachidonic– contains 4 double bonds

Good sources of unsaturated fats are safflower, peanut, olive and grape seed oil. Average Americans now consumes over 50lb of saturated fat/yr, or approximately 600 cal/day, mostly from animal sources. The greater consumption of saturated fat, the greater the chance of coronary heart disease (CHD).

Saturated fat is popular with commercial enterprises because it is resistant to oxidation, and does not go rancid easily. It also stores well at room temperature because it is solid. However not all saturated fat is bad. Drugs such as epinephrine (adrenaline), glucagon, growth hormone, and steroids mobilize fat and increase their metabolism. **During prolonged exercise 80% of the energy used is derived from fat, a good reason for exercise.** Just 1-4 hours of moderate exercise, causes a 70% mobilization of fatty acids. Unsaturated fats are readily oxidized and go rancid quickly. Therefore you should refrigerate them after opening. 10-15% of your daily food intake should consist of fat. Less than 30% should be saturated fat.

Metabolism: Metabolism is the sum total of all body reactions, and it slows down with an increase in age. As the graph below shows, a 1% decrease occurs per year past the age of 20 years. Male hormone levels also drop with age, as do estrogen levels in females. Obesity and overweight have become the main public health problem in the United States. Over 60% of all adults are considered overweight, and 30% of adults are considered obsess. The rate of childhood obesity has become almost epidemic.

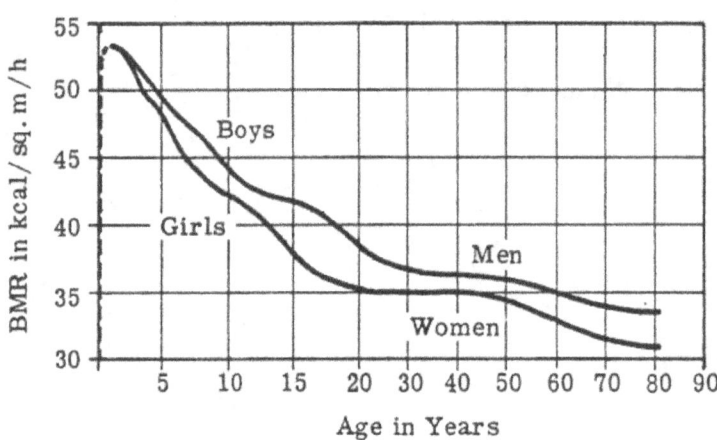

Change in BMR with age (from Mitchell, 1962)

Body Composition: Here are some statistics on the body fat averages of American men and women.

Women - Average American woman is 27.0%

 Lean -19.9% or less

Average – 20.0-25.0%

Overweight – 25.0 – 29.9%

Obese – Greater than 30.0%

Men - Average American Male is 17.0%

 Lean – 9.9% or less

Average – 10.0 – 14.9%

Overweight – 15.0 – 19.9%

Obese – greater than 20.0%

These body fat averages would make Europeans shudder. Women are normally "fatter" than men, and also breast development is about 3%. However too many of us are overweight. What can be done? Diet and workout!!!!!!! Our diet should be proportioned as follows:

60-70% carbohydrate, 15-20% protein, 10-15% fats, primarily unsaturated fats

Vitamins and Minerals

<table>
<tr>
<td colspan="2">Fat Soluble Vitamins: Require the presence of bile for proper absorption. Any defect in fat absorption could lead to vitamin deficiencies.</td>
</tr>
<tr>
<td>A</td>
<td>

- Nutritional factors – vitamin A, provitamin, alpha/ beta/gamma carotenes, and ryptoxanthine.
- Conversions of the precursors occur in the liver and the wall of the small intestine.
- Fish liver oil contains vitamin A and its precusors.
- Involved in the maintenance of the epithelial tissues.
- Vitamin A-aldehyde functions in the ada[tational changes of the retinato light and dark.
- Deficiency can cause: retarded growth, xeropthalmia (spectacle eye), impaired epithelial tissues, and night-blindness.
- Contained in milk, eggs, vegetables, liver oils, liver, and glandular organs.
- Can be stored in the liver – **A DANGER.**
-
</td>
</tr>
<tr>
<td>D</td>
<td>

- Necessary for absorption of calcium from the intestine, and for reabsorption of phosphates in the kidney.
- Needed for normal bone growth and for normal respiratory function.
- Obtained through UVlight, irradiation of ergosterol.
-
</td>
</tr>
<tr>
<td>E</td>
<td>

- Tocopherols
- Primary function is as an antioxidant.
-
</td>
</tr>
<tr>
<td>K</td>
<td>

- Possesses anti-hemorrhagic reactions
- Involved with the blood clotting mechanism.
-
</td>
</tr>
</table>

Water Soluble Vitamins	
B-complex	• Oxidation-reduction reactions. • Red blood cell formation. •
Ascorbic acid – Vitamin C	• Active in tissue respiration, general resistance to disease, and formation of intercellular cement / collagen formation. • Deficiencies cause bone wounds to heal slowly and capillary fragility. • The adrenal cortex contains large quantities of vitamin C, which suggest its use in the formation of steroid hormones. • A liberal daily intake of vitamin C is recommended throughout life. • It is the least resistant of the vitamins: labile destroyed by heat, damaged by drying, oxidized in alkaline solutions, destroyed in iron and copper utensils, destroyed by storage, canning, and cooking.

Minerals – 40% of our body weight is primarily in the skeletal system.	
Calcium	<ul><li>Constituent of protoplasm and body fluids.</li><li>99% is located in the bones and teeth.</li><li>Important in permeability of cell membranes. Excitability of muscles, normal heart action, nerve activity and blood clotting.</li><li>**Calcium deficiency in the United States is a real problem.**</li></ul>
Phosphorus	<ul><li>Particularly important in nerve and muscle tissue.</li><li>80% found in teeth and bones.</li><li>Important in the absorption of carbohydrates in the intestine, phospholipids, phosphocreatine, phosphorylated intermediates.</li><li>Important in the absorption of vitamin D</li><li>Acid-base balance.</li><li>Found in milk, cheese, meat, liver, kidney, fish and eggs.</li></ul>
Iron	<ul><li>Found in hemoglobin, myoglobin of skeletal muscle, cytochrome and enzyme systems.</li><li>Found in tissues as ferritin.</li><li>Found as protein bound iron in the liver as a storage form.</li><li>Essential for the utilization of iron.</li><li>Contained in whole-grains, egg-yolk, beef, fruits, vegetables, fish, oysters, and beans.</li><li>12-12mg of iron in the body.</li></ul>
Copper	<ul><li>Involved in hemoglobin formation.</li><li>Involved in many enzyme systems.</li><li>2 mg required daily.</li><li>Contained in liver, fruits, nuts, vegetables, and beans.</li></ul>

Magnesium	<ul><li>Serves as a cofactor in the metabolism of glucose, pyruvic acid, and ATP.</li><li>229 mg required daily.</li><li>Found in meat and vegetables.</li><li>Excessive amounts can cause depression of nerve cell impulses.</li><li>Used as a tranquilizer for fish.</li></ul>
Potassium	<ul><li>Involved in nerve transmission, skeletal muscle contraction, and cardiac muscle contraction.</li><li>Depletion causes the immediate malfunction of the heart.</li><li>Require 2-4 mg daily.</li><li>Found in vegetables, fruit, and meat.</li></ul>
Iodine	<ul><li>Used in the synthesis of thyroxin in the thyroid gland.</li><li>Should intake 0.15-0.30mg daily.</li><li>Found in milk, vegetables, fruit, fish, and shellfish.</li></ul>
Cobalt	<ul><li>Essential for red-blood cell and B_{12} formation.</li></ul>
Manganese	<ul><li>Activates important enzymes.</li><li>Ubiquitous, found in many foods.</li></ul>
Zinc	<ul><li>Found in many enzyme systems.</li><li>Ubiquitous.</li></ul>
Fluorine	<ul><li>Found in tooth and bone structure.</li></ul>
Trace minerals	<ul><li>Cesium, strontium, and boron.</li></ul>

Conclusion

Now that we have covered physical fitness, digestion and nutrition, I believe that you have all the information you need to design your own fitness and nutrition program, a program you can follow throughout your life with a little modification as needed.   I am not offering a miracle diet, or an exercise program that will have you losing 30 lbs. in 30 days. But I am offering a solid understanding of diet and exercise that can help you develop a sound way of approaching your health and fitness for the rest of your life. I look at diet as a 4 letter word, and so should you. Hard work and proper eating will help you succeed in maintaining fitness for life.

The main point I would like to make is that you can maintain a healthy life style no matter what challenges you may face (aging, health issues etc.). I am facing both aging (I am 70 years old), and health issues (I was diagnosed with multiple myeloma 8 years ago), and yet I exercise every day at home and in the pool, and I eat well. By eating 5 small meals a day, based on the schedule below, I am eating wisely and not stressing out my digestive system. Of course I avoid "junk or fast" foods.

60-70% carbohydrate

15-20% protein

10-15% fats, primarily unsaturated fats

Yes! Anyone can start an exercise program, and anyone can improve their nutrition using this book as a guide to develop a sensible eating/exercising program. I believe that we can improve our fitness, and nutrition no matter what age we are. There is no secret, just hard work, proper nutrition, and making the decision to get started – and stay with it! I hope this book has provided the tools to allow you to design your own program.

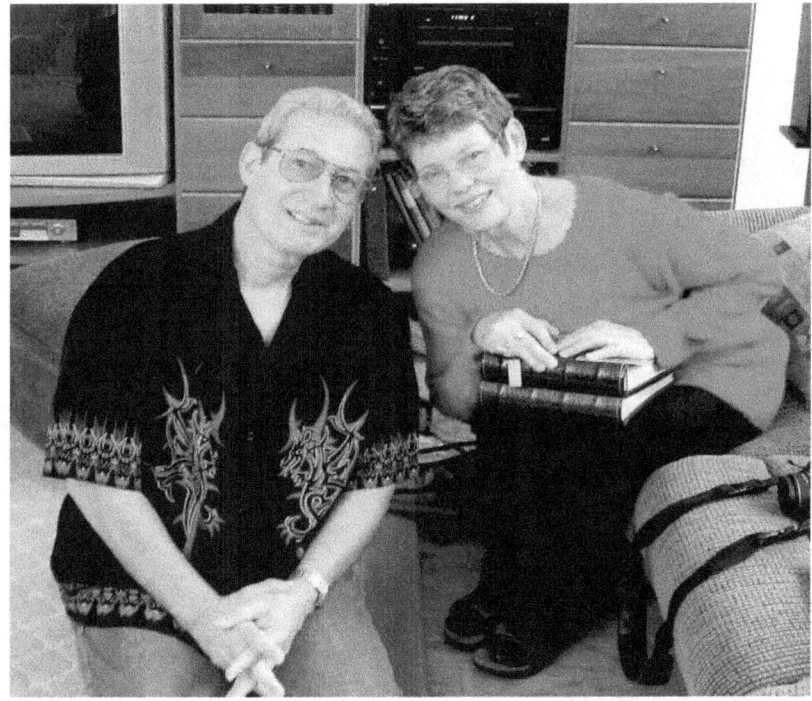

Looking Forward to Many More Years!
Stan Morey & Gery Morey in their late 60's

About the Author

Stanley Morey, Ph.D. is an accomplished author, writing many books in the bodybuilding and nutrition areas. He received his B.S. from the University of Tampa, attended J. Hillis Miller Medical School in Gainesville, and the University of South Florida, in Tampa. He received his Ph. D. from the California Institute of Technology, Pacific College in 1972 in Physiology. He was also a competitive bodybuilder for many years, winning many local and regional competitions.

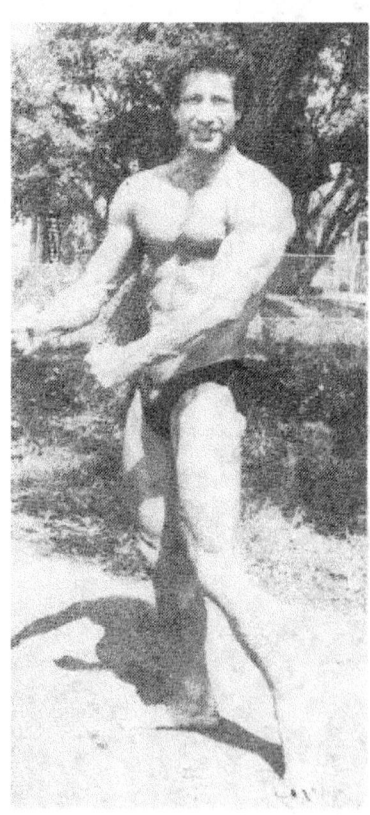

www.ingramcontent.com/pod-product-compliance
Lightning Source LLC
Chambersburg PA
CBHW080921290526
45795CB00007BA/2602